CAREER AS A

NURSE EDUCATOR

TEACHING THE NEXT GENERATION OF NURSES

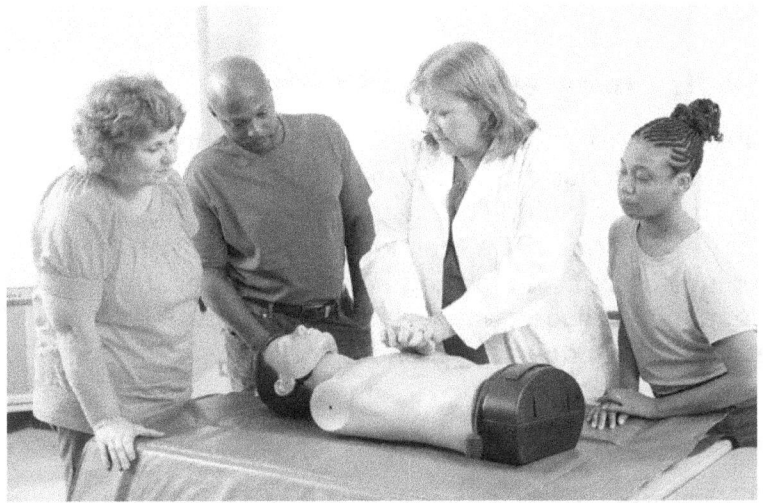

THERE HAS NEVER BEEN A BETTER TIME to consider a career in the nursing field. The nursing shortage in the US has been worsening for several years and there appears to be no end in sight. The demand for nursing services has been growing steadily due to an aging population, greater access to health insurance, and an increased emphasis on preventive care. As a result, the country will need 1.13 million more nurses by 2022, according to the

American Nurses Association.

However, there is a problem. The healthcare industry cannot keep up with the growing demand for new nurses because there are not enough nurse educators to train them. Without teachers, schools cannot accept new students. According to the National League for Nursing survey, more than half of all nursing schools turn qualified applicants away each year. That means there is tremendous opportunity for nurse educators who are prepared to fill the many open faculty positions. Anyone who chooses to become a nurse educator will most likely have a choice of employers.

What is a nurse educator?

Nurse educators are registered nurses who teach and train aspiring nurses. Most have a high level of expertise gained from working in direct patient care as nurses themselves. They share their knowledge and skills with nursing students in teaching hospitals, universities, community colleges, and vocational schools. Job responsibilities do vary depending on the employer, but generally nurse educators:

Develop lesson plans

Give lectures

Create and conduct exams

Oversee student nurses' clinical practice

Evaluate students' progress

Act as advisors and serve as role models

The courses nurse educators teach may cover general nursing topics or focus on areas of specialization, such as acute care or pediatric health. After gaining some teaching experience, they may be asked to create new courses or programs, write or review textbooks, develop continuing education programs for working nurses, or give lectures at professional nursing conferences. They may also advance to administrative roles, such as managing nurse education programs, or eventually becoming the dean of a nursing school.

An advanced education is needed to become a nurse educator. There are several choices but the most common is a Master of Science in Nursing degree (MSN). MSN programs are available in traditional classroom settings and online. They are open to students with a bachelor's degree, and it does not have to be a nursing degree. Aspiring nurse educators who want to advance into academic administration or research will need to earn a Doctor of Philosophy degree (PhD). A PhD in nursing can also be extremely valuable when applying for the best nurse educator jobs.

Once on the job, nurse educators must continue learning and stay on the leading edge of clinical practice by reading professional journals, attending seminars and conferences, and practicing at least part time in a clinical setting. This is extremely important, not only for their own teaching career, but for the success of their students.

Nurse education offers a high degree of professional satisfaction. Helping future nurses learn and grow is reportedly the most rewarding aspect of the work. Other benefits of the career include access to cutting-edge knowledge and research, an intellectually stimulating workplace, opportunities for advancement, and good work/life balance. However you look at it, becoming a nurse educator is an excellent career move.

WHAT YOU CAN DO NOW

BECOMING A NURSE EDUCATOR requires a considerable amount of education. In high school, make sure you take the classes that you will need to be admitted to a college with a nursing program. Admission requirements vary, but generally you will need to take four years of math and science classes. Take Advanced Placement (AP) classes whenever possible and keep your GPA as high as you can.

Join HOSA-Future Health Professionals if it is available at your school. This is an instructional program designed to prepare students for a future in health sciences. In your junior year, ask your counselor to help you become a teacher's assistant (TA) to get a sense of what teaching is like.

Contact the colleges that interest you and visit if possible. Most schools have information on their websites about application deadlines, which entrance exams are required (SAT, ACT, or others), and whether there is a waiting list for the nursing program. Keep in mind that nursing programs have an additional admission process. They are very competitive and only a fraction of the applicants are admitted. The best way to ensure you are one of the lucky ones is to keep your grades up. Admissions are typically based on both high school GPAs as well as college entrance exam scores.

Outside of school, you can prepare by taking a first aid and CPR class or going to nursing camp. To get some real world nursing experience, volunteer in a hospital or clinic, or get a summer or part-time job in the healthcare field. Although it is fine to answer phones or do other tasks that let you see nurses in action, the best situation is one that allows you to work directly with patients. This is possible in nursing homes and Veterans Administration (VA) hospitals. Volunteering in these settings provides valuable experience and will boost your chances of gaining admission to nursing school.

HISTORY OF THE PROFESSION

NURSING HAS EXISTED FOR THOUSANDS OF YEARS, slowly evolving over the course of history.

As a distinct profession, it is believed to have taken root around 300 AD while the Roman Empire was determined to erect a hospital in every town under its rule. During the Middle Ages, the concept of professional nursing spread across Europe and eventually around the world. It was during this time that the nurse's role within the hospital environment expanded to include many of the various duties that nurses still perform today. Although the framework of modern nursing began to progress during the 10th and 11th centuries, it did not start to take shape until the 19th century.

In the mid-1850s, during the Crimean War, the renowned Florence Nightingale changed the very nature of the nursing profession forever. Deaths on the battlefield were all too common. Lack of general hygiene led to fatal infections from even the most minor injuries. With aid from the British government, Nightingale was able to establish sanitary conditions for patients, both on the battlefield and in a nearby hospital. As a result, the death rate from infections dropped dramatically in a very short period of time.

In 1860, Nightingale founded the first nursing school in London. The Florence Nightingale School for Nurses provided a blueprint for other schools to open and provide formal training and education to aspiring nurses. One of those schools, the New England Hospital for Women, became the first nursing school to open in the United States. In 1873, it graduated its first nurse trainee after she completed the one-year program. The school was based on the Florence Nightingale model, which focused on evidence-based practice and systematic patient data collection within the hospital environment.

The 1893 Chicago World's Fair introduced 26 million people to Cracker Jacks, zippers, dishwashers, and aerosol spray paint. It also hosted the first true global meeting of nurses, all of whom advocated for higher education for nurses. Florence Nightingale did not attend, but she did submit her most significant White Paper. She and her colleagues made a compelling case for standardized higher education that would replace the model of the time in which most nurses trained by serving as apprentices in hospitals. Their pleas were heard, and later that year the American Society of Superintendents of Training Schools for Nurses (later renamed the National League for Nursing) was founded. As the first professional nursing organization, it established the first standard curriculum for nursing schools. The enthusiasm for higher education for nurses got a boost from many states that began to pass legislation requiring licensure based on the demonstration of professional knowledge and skills.

In 1923, Yale University opened the first autonomous school of nursing outside the hospital environment. The Yale School of Nursing had its own dean, faculty, budget and degree. More importantly, it provided training that was based on broadly relevant, quality education, rather than the service needs of a hospital.

Despite these milestones, nursing education developed very haphazardly until the 1950s. Throughout the first half of the 20th century, the training for most American nurses consisted of on-the-job training in hospitals. Some hospitals offered "diplomas," but they were meaningless outside the particular issuing hospital. Nursing students were simply a source of free labor that hospitals were reluctant to give up. The training itself was spotty at best. It was common for the irregularly scheduled classes to be cancelled when students were needed to work in the wards.

After repeated calls for nursing schools to be relocated to universities, advances in science and technology finally forced the issue. Keeping up with the rapid changes in healthcare delivery became too much for hospitals. At first, the universities offered only four-year bachelor's degree programs, but they quickly realized they could not produce nurses fast enough to meet the demand.

In the early 1950s, the first two-year associate degree nursing program was created at the Adelphi College School of Nursing in New York state. The purpose of the program was to provide adequate technical training to meet immediate demand while other nurses were going through the full four-year training. Now there were three ways to become a Registered Nurse (RN): through a two-year associate degree, a three-year diploma program, or four-year baccalaureate program. The American Nurses Association lobbied for four-year programs, asserting that higher educational standards were in the best interests of patients. The Nurse Training Act of 1964 aimed to phase out hospital diploma programs and required that all nursing education should take place in institutions of higher education. It also infused a tremendous amount of funding into collegiate programs, initiated graduate studies, and advanced practice programs.

Still, hospitals were slow to comply and serious movement into the university system did not occur until the 1980s. Technology, again, played a major role in the shift. The first generation of human body simulators with specialized features were introduced in nursing classrooms. One of the first simulations, named Surgeon, was actually able to simulate operating on an aortic aneurysm. All but the largest teaching hospitals shifted their focus to the care of their patients and left the education of nurses to the academics.

For more than a century now, reports on nursing education have pushed for higher education and greater responsibilities for nurses. Nursing education continues to evolve, promote higher standards, and further the advancement of nursing as a profession. Today, universities and community colleges are vital partners in the healthcare profession. Their training programs and the nurse educators who present them are challenging future nurses to develop critical thinking skills, utilize cutting edge technology, and assume leadership roles wherever they practice.

The nursing profession has come a long way over the millennia. Once seen as inexpensive healthcare workers, nurses are now recognized as the highly educated, respected professionals they are. The field of nursing education has evolved from the on-the-spot, haphazard acquisition of skills on the battlefield to an intellectually demanding array of abilities learned in the classroom, on the internet, and at the bedside.

WHERE YOU WILL WORK

NURSE EDUCATORS CAN BE FOUND WORKING wherever there are nursing classes. That includes educational institutions that offer nursing degree or certificate programs, such as colleges and universities, community colleges, and trade and vocational schools. Even some high schools offer nursing education. However, the majority of jobs are in colleges and universities.

A smaller number of nurse educators work in hospitals and long-term care facilities. These are usually larger facilities that have their own training programs for nurses. Nurse educators may also work in large private medical practices training other nurses, in schools teaching children about nursing, and in online tutoring through distance learning programs. A very small number of nurse educators work in research, which may be part of a university's doctoral program or a private consulting firm.

The primary work setting is the college campus, but there are many different kinds of environments. They may be located in urban, suburban, small town, or rural areas. They may be private universities or public community colleges. They may be associated with a vocational school, but situated inside a teaching hospital.

A nurse educator's day is divided between the classroom giving lectures and in an office. Office time is spent advising students, preparing lessons, grading papers, and handling other administrative duties. There are also periodic faculty meetings held somewhere on campus. It is common for nurse educators to supervise students in clinical settings, which may be in a nearby hospital or other healthcare facility.

Nurse educators who work in schools typically teach during the nine-month academic year and either take the summers off or do something else until the next school term begins. Those who work in hospitals may work year-round, but have nursing duties in addition to teaching. Nurse educators in general work regular daytime hours. They do not have to work the usual 12-hour or overnight shifts that clinical nurses do.

THE WORK YOU WILL DO

THE JOB OF THE NURSE EDUCATOR IS TO TEACH. For most nurse educators, this means teaching students to become nurses. This may take place in a clinical environment or an academic setting. The clinical environment would likely be a hospital or other medical facility, while the academic setting is a school, such as a university, community college, or vocational school. It is often a combination of both.

A nurse educator's day is typically divided between lecturing in the classroom and overseeing students practice what they have learned in a real world setting such as a nearby hospital, community clinic, or long-term care facility. Classroom instruction includes courses related to the scientific and medical sides of nursing, but there is a lot more to nursing than scientific facts. Good quality nursing involves a variety of intangibles, such as regulations, medical ethics, professionalism, respect for privacy, emotional balance, and best practices for interacting with patients.

Outside the classroom, nurse educators supervise students as they apply what they have learned in hands-on simulations. Some schools provide clinical labs where students can perform basic tasks such as administering medications, taking vital signs, or changing dressings under the supervision of the nurse educator. Once students have mastered some basic skills, they move into real life clinical settings, where they perform actual nursing tasks. The nurse educator continues to oversee and monitor the progress of students as they work with patients.

At the most basic level, a nurse educator's job is to teach future nurses how to provide patient care. The job, however, is rarely as simple as that sounds. Depending on their role and the dictates of their employer, general tasks may include any or all of the following.

Design and implement lesson plans

Lecture on a number of scientific and healthcare topics

Assign homework

Develop and administer exams

Grade papers and evaluate student progress

Oversee student lab and clinical work

Promote discussions among students

Serve as student adviser on academic issues

Mentor students regarding career paths

Participate in professional associations

Speak at nursing conferences

It is vital that nurse educators stay abreast of evolving nursing techniques and emerging technological developments. Teaching outdated information is never acceptable. Nurse educators are often asked to update or redesign old courses, or even create new ones. In order to keep up, nurse educators need to be students themselves. They read professional journals and study to maintain a current knowledge base. They also continue to work part time as nurses to keep their skills fresh.

Some nurse educators do not teach nursing students at all. Instead, they work with patients, which often means instructing individuals who do not have a medical background. They may work one-on-one with individual patients, such as those dealing with long-term conditions like diabetes. They may also teach classes for family members, such as those who have relatives with cancer or

Alzheimer's. Patient education may be provided in the home, but is more commonly organized in a hospital setting. Some nurse educators teach the general public about health issues. This may mean a one-time engagement to lead a first aid or CPR course at a community center or speaking at a retiree club about how to deal with a current health danger such as a flu epidemic or the importance of getting a shingles vaccination.

Teaching in a Hospital

Nurse education used to exist primarily in hospitals, where the nurse educators were expected to provide nursing services while training incoming nursing staff. Today's nursing educators do still teach nursing students in hospitals, but mostly in teaching hospitals. These are large facilities that are universities and medical centers combined, such as Mayo Clinic, UCSF Medical Center, and Cleveland Clinic.

As faculty members in teaching hospitals, nurse educators have the usual responsibilities of creating lesson plans, lecturing, supervising students in clinical assignments, and generally making sure students are developing good nursing skills. In addition, they may be expected to help update nursing policies, train new staff members, track the continuing education of nurses, and monitor certifications. Some nurse educators have even heftier responsibilities like maintaining budgets, tracking the outcomes of new programs (quality control), participating in physician-directed research projects, preparing and overseeing orientation for new nurses, and developing training courses including major segments of curricula.

In a non-teaching hospital, the exact duties of the nurse educator depend on the particular hospital's needs. Many are involved in the training of new hires. Others are focused on patient care and instruction. A nurse educator in this role often develops new patient education programs for the hospital and oversees the running of these projects.

The Academic Setting

Many nurse educators teach at a college or university, instructing students who are working toward undergraduate or graduate degrees in nursing. In some cases, they teach refresher courses for nurses who want to return to their careers after being out of the field for some time.

College faculty positions include adjunct (part-time instructor), clinical instructor, lecturer, assistant professor, associate professor, and full professor. In addition to the usual teaching tasks, faculty members sometimes act as student advisers, perform peer reviews, lecture at annual nursing conferences, and write grant proposals for nonprofit community health education projects. There are also a variety of administrative tasks that may be included in the nurse educator's job description.

Nurse educators in the academic setting usually have the choice of whether to continue to also practice nursing. Many do so part time in local hospitals to maintain their clinical skills.

At the university level, nurse educators are often required to participate in research studies and present the results at nursing conferences. In some cases, the information that results from the research is incorporated into new nursing program curricula. Nurse educators may also be expected to publish their own research from time to time.

Advancement

Nurse educators with advanced education and solid experience can move into a variety of roles. In the hospital setting, one of the common first steps out of the classroom is taking charge of continuing education of nursing staff. In collaboration with hospital administrators, they study the healthcare delivery needs of the institution and then determine the best educational resources for nursing staff to meet those needs. They may create development manuals and training guides that incorporate new procedures and systems, and facilitate the associated training. They may also be involved in employee evaluations and remediation.

In the academic setting, experienced nurse educators may advance into an administrative position and possibly even become dean of the nursing program. Depending on the individual's role, job responsibilities may include consulting with instructors to develop new or improved courses, or even entire nursing programs. They would then develop budgets, secure funding, hire necessary staff, and supervise the implementation of the programs. The dean of a nursing program does all of this and more. It is the dean's responsibility to ensure that the content of the nursing program is up to date and relevant. This usually entails seeking input and feedback from regular interaction with the healthcare facilities within the community.

There are also numerous roles that experienced nurse educators can pursue outside of direct care education. Some have an organizational focus, such as corporate health program management or clinical research coordination. Others arise from new changes in the continuously evolving field of healthcare. For example, a forward-thinking nurse educator might want to be part of innovative solutions to domestic health reform or the global healthcare system. At the government level, that might include setting public policy. Some nurse educators might prefer to work behind the scenes on less exciting, yet very necessary, academic areas such as informatics (the science of storing, processing, and retrieving health information). Others are motivated to add to the body of nursing knowledge and choose to get involved in research at independent laboratories.

STORIES OF NURSE EDUCATORS

I Teach Nurses in a Traditional University Setting

"My students are current nurses who want to advance their careers. After graduation, they will become nurse practitioners or clinical specialists in areas such as trauma, cardiac surgery, or neurology.

All of my lessons start with a lecture, but there is much more to my classes. Textbooks and lectures are still the basis of nursing education, but I supplement each lesson with Internet research, videos, PowerPoint presentations, and other electronic media. Most importantly, I oversee clinical instruction. This is an area that has changed a lot over the years. Technology now plays a major role. For example, we have life-like simulation dummies that provide very real opportunities to practice skills like central line insertion. Can you imagine trying to put an endotracheal tube (breathing tube) into a live patient's mouth and get it positioned in the airway the first time? Now, instead of worrying about harming the patient, the student can focus on perfecting the skill. Students can even simulate various scenarios that cover abnormal symptoms so they're prepared to make quick decisions when faced with atypical situations.

Perhaps the most important part of my job is keeping up with what is going on in current healthcare practice and adjust my lesson plans accordingly. Over the past decade, for instance, the number of older patients has been growing steadily. It is the main reason more nurses are needed. To address this fact, I incorporated gerontology into the curriculum. I don't just teach about the common diseases of aging though. I instruct my students how to approach and interact with aging patients and their families. I have student actors come in and simulate typical needs and problems of the elderly while my students practice responding.

My advice for future nurse educators is to never stop learning. To do a good job, it is necessary to also be the student. Keeping up with changes and advances in the field is vital. You can do this by reading and attending seminars, but I think teachers should also continue doing some clinical nursing in order to remain relevant."

I Teach Nurses to Work in Obstetrics

"I teach obstetrical nursing courses within the four-year bachelor's degree nursing program. The study of pregnancy and childbirth has always been my passion so I am thrilled to play a role in the development of the next generation of nurses.

My career started in high school, when I landed my first job as a nursing assistant. I went on to nursing school and after graduation worked in the maternity ward of my hometown hospital. My supervisor noticed that I tended to jump in and take on leadership roles. She suggested I put my talents to work as a teacher. I completed a master's degree in clinical nursing, took extra courses in curriculum development, and obtained three professional certifications related to obstetrics. The certifications weren't required to become a nurse educator, but the work I did to earn them really helped me do a better job of designing and teaching courses and seminars.

About 20 percent of my time is spent in the classroom giving lectures. I spend much more time overseeing the clinical work my students do in nearby hospitals where they assist doctors attending to pregnant women before, during, and after delivery. I also create exams, read and grade papers, and evaluate student presentations. To keep up with new developments, I read professional journals, attend nursing conferences, and participate in various educational committees.

My advice to nurses thinking of getting into teaching is to get as much education as you can. Get a master's degree, and if possible, go for a doctoral degree. That is what the best jobs require. Make sure you spend time gaining some clinical experience in a variety of settings and then focus on a specialized area that interests you. Having a specialization will make you even more desirable as a job candidate. Along the way, wherever you go, network. Networking is very important in this profession. It's how most of us get our jobs. I landed my first faculty position through a recommendation from one of my colleagues that I met at a continuing education seminar. I wouldn't even have known there was an opening if it hadn't been for that contact keeping in touch."

I Am an Adjunct Assistant Professor

"I chose to be a nurse because I wanted to help people and do my part to make the world a little better. For me, nursing was the ideal choice to realize that goal. I chose to be a nurse educator for the very same reasons. Now I not only help patients, but I also help young nurses realize their career and life goals. It is rewarding to be a part of that process.

When I was ready to make the transition to teaching, I wanted to stay close to home. At the time, there weren't any full-time positions nearby, but there were adjunct positions available. In fact, I was offered two adjunct positions – one at a local community college and one at a university with an easy commute. I chose the university and have been an adjunct in the associate degree nursing program for three years now.

I've been offered the opportunity to take a full-time faculty position, but it turns out I enjoy the flexibility of teaching part time. I teach four foundation classes, which doesn't require much prep time. When I'm not teaching, I put in about four hours a day in clinical practice at the local hospital. So I am able to help prepare the next generation of nurses while still caring for patients. Seems like a win-win to me.

If I were to consider taking a full-time faculty position, I would need to return to school for a doctoral degree. I might do that someday, but for now, I enjoy many of the benefits of being a faculty member without the investment. I have been able to collaborate with faculty members on manuscripts and proposals. I've been a guest speaker at several nursing conferences. I'm involved in community health education programs, and I've even worked on some cutting edge research projects. I think new graduates should take adjunct opportunities seriously. It's an alternative that has more to offer than simply being a stepping stone to better jobs."

PERSONAL QUALIFICATIONS

TEACHERS WILL TELL YOU THAT THEY DO what they do because they love it. Nurse educators are no different. The best nurse educators are those who are the most passionate about education. They live to prepare their students to be the best nurses they can be.

Make no mistake, teaching is not an easy job. If you do not enjoy teaching, it is not the career for you. If you are ready to meet the day-to-day challenges of the classroom, you will thrive. Passion in all aspects of teaching is the number one characteristic of all good nurse educators. There are other traits, though, that successful nurse educators share.

Communications Skills

Good nurse educators are able to explain complex concepts in clear language that novices can understand. When a student does not understand the first time, the teacher is able to rephrase the message to meet the learning style of the student. Teachers are confident in their knowledge, possess strong leadership qualities, and have no fear of public speaking. The best nurse educators have the ability to quickly build rapport with people – a particularly helpful skill when managing difficult students.

Adaptability

Change is a fact of life in the nursing world. Whenever changes occur in clinical settings, nurse educators must incorporate those changes into their lesson plans. Adaptation is a key skill even when there are no external forces at work. No two students are alike. Classrooms are filled with students of various levels of ability, learning styles, and backgrounds. This is one of the biggest challenges for nurse educators. They cannot simply use the same template for every group. They need to anticipate making changes to meet the needs of all the students, not just the majority.

Dedication

It takes time and hard work to become a nurse. Some students may waver under the mental, emotional, and physical demands of the profession. Teachers who are clearly dedicated to nursing, and to the success of the future nurses under their tutelage, set a good example for those who are struggling. Reiterating the rewards of dedication into classroom discussions can inspire students to go the distance.

Patience

Nurse educators often have to remind themselves that producing good nurses takes time. Having patience with yourself and your students is essential throughout the process. Patience can overcome discouragement, fear, and frustration on both sides of the lectern. Every teacher has a personal way of demonstrating patience. Whatever techniques are applied to teaching can be imparted to students so they, too, will be able to deal with challenges in a disciplined, calm manner.

Positive Attitude

A nurse educator experiences many ups and downs. Molding the minds of future nurses is a rewarding experience, but along the way there will be tedious paperwork, big egos, academic bureaucracy, and bad tempers to deal with. A nurse educator with a positive attitude can cope with everyday setbacks in stride. Add a good sense of humor and even the worst day can bring moments of levity and lower the stress levels of you and your students.

ATTRACTIVE FEATURES

NURSE EDUCATORS REPORT A HIGH DEGREE of satisfaction with their career choice. They cite an intellectually stimulating workplace, access to cutting-edge research, and the opportunity to collaborate with all kinds of health professionals as the top reasons for loving what they do. They also enjoy better than average pay, flexible work scheduling, autonomy, and the chance to wear something more stylish than a uniform.

Other benefits of careers in nursing education include:

A Rosy Job Outlook

It is common knowledge that there is a nursing shortage, but most people do not realize that the main reason is the lack of nurse educators to prepare the next generation. The need for nurse educators is so great, thousands of qualified nursing school applicants are turned away each year because there are insufficient numbers of teachers to teach them. As a result, nurse educators have excellent job prospects with future advancement opportunities and a level of job security most people can only dream of.

The Best of Nursing

Nurse educators have dedicated years to nursing because they love it. They do not necessarily love the 12-hour shifts, working on holidays and weekends, and being on their feet until their bodies ache. Nurse educators are still in the hospital, but they do minimal care and they are not fully responsible for patients. Most of the time they work in an office or classroom, or supervising student nurses for an hour at a time. The hours are shorter and there is a good chance of creating a good work-life balance.

A Variety of Work Environments

Nurses have few options when it comes to work settings. They are either in a hospital, clinic, physician's office, or some other healthcare facility where they interact directly with patients. Nurse educators on the other hand, can choose where and how they work. They can teach in schools or in a clinical setting or both. They can teach and still care for patients, or focus solely on teaching. They are needed everywhere so they can move to wherever they like. They can even teach from anywhere in the world, using technology.

Rewards of Teaching

Nurse educators play a critical role in the healthcare field. They are the leaders who shape the future of nursing by training the nurses who will care for patients long into the future. Along the way, they contribute to the body of nursing knowledge, inspire future nurses to be the best they can be, and generally make the profession of nursing better. In return, nurse educators are respected for the role they play and are remembered by students long after they launch their nursing careers.

UNATTRACTIVE ASPECTS

NURSE EDUCATORS TEACH BECAUSE THEY LOVE IT, not because it is easy. It is great to be able to change a career path without changing careers, but it takes several years of advanced education to make that change. Plus, the education needs to cover two areas: advanced nursing concepts and teaching skills.

Getting a job as a nurse educator is relatively easy, but once on the job there are challenges. There is constant paperwork, lesson preparation, and other tasks outside the classroom. That means you cannot leave work at work, but usually have much to do at home after hours. Those who teach in schools are often surprised by the unexpected demands on their time. In the university setting, there are often research and publishing requirements. They may need to write grant proposals to cover funding for new research projects or serve on academic committees. In the hospital arena, they may be expected to actively participate in professional conferences or speak at seminars. They can say goodbye to 12-hour shifts on their feet, but addressing all their responsibilities within eight hours may prove difficult.

Nurse educators are paid well, but considering the high level of education required and the many hours spent preparing and grading lessons, salaries could be better. In fact, the average salary for a nurse educator is lower than that of other nurses with advanced degrees. A nurse practitioner, for example, earns nearly $10,000 a year more than a nurse educator with the same level of education. In the academic setting, professors of nursing earn less than their non-nursing faculty colleagues.

EDUCATION AND TRAINING

AN ADVANCED EDUCATION IS needed to become a nurse educator. It could be a Master of Science in Nursing degree (MSN) or doctoral degree in nursing (PhD), each of which require a chosen clinical specialization. MSN programs are available in traditional classroom settings and online. The coursework builds on the undergraduate curriculum of a nursing degree program. An associate degree or bachelor's degree in a field other than nursing can be used to enter an accelerated program for a Bachelor of Science (BSN) before pursuing an MSN.

The more popular path is a master's degree and/or post-graduate certificate program created specifically for nurse educators, such as the MS in Nursing Education or the MS in Nursing with a Concentration in Nursing Education. These programs are considered the standard for nurse educators because they are designed to meet eligibility requirements for the Certified Nurse Educator (CNE) exam.

All nurse education programs introduce nurses to teaching methods and curricula design theory. Typical courses include:

Education Strategies in Nursing

Nursing Curriculum Development and Evaluation

Education and Assessment in Nursing

Instructional Design

Principles of Adult Learning

Principles of Teaching and Learning

Instructional Technology

There are also courses in healthcare policy, ethics, advanced health promotion, and nursing and public policy. These courses provide a good foundation for potential advancement in academia.

Nurse educators are expected to have a much broader knowledge base than the average registered nurse. In addition to education courses, they study advanced concepts in pathophysiology and nursing research, evolution of nursing theory, advanced health assessment, and the newest pharmacologic applications.

Extensive clinical nursing experience in a hospital or other medical facility is a must. Nursing educators do more than give lectures. They teach clinical skills and oversee students as they practice what they have learned in nearby hospitals. In addition, nurse educators are expected to keep up with changes in the clinical environment. They usually stay up to date with the newest medical technologies and evolving nursing practices by continuing to work part time with patients.

Doctoral Level

Aspiring nurse educators who want to advance in academia will need to earn a doctoral degree. There are several choices to consider, depending on one's goals. A PhD is required for any kind of research and a general PhD in Nursing is fine for research professors. Those who aspire to become nursing program directors, however, will need a PhD in Higher Education Administration. There are also Doctor of Nursing Philosophy programs that focus on leadership and public policy issues.

Future nurse educators who know early on that they want to earn a PhD should look for schools that offer bachelor's to PhD degree programs. There are many colleges and universities offering these programs for nurses with bachelor's degrees. What sets them apart is the focus on doctoral preparation while the student skips the master's degree.

There are also programs for students with non-nursing undergraduate degrees, such as the MSN/PhD Dual Degree, that helps fill in the vital nursing education that may be missing.

Certification

Certification in this field is voluntary, but highly encouraged as it demonstrates advanced knowledge and skills in the specialty area of nursing education. The Certified Nurse Education (CNE) designation is available through the National League for Nursing (NLN). There are two levels of certification available, but generally, eligibility criteria include an active RN license in the US, an advanced degree in nursing education, and a minimum two years of full-time teaching experience. Depending on the level, experience may be substituted for education level or vice versa. There is also an examination covering all aspects of teaching responsibilities, methodologies, leadership, and student development.

Nurse educators can also obtain certification for teaching in a specialized area related to a single disease or type of disorder. There are dozens of specialty areas to choose from. A few of the most popular include diabetes, oncology, pediatrics, acute care, cardiology, mental health, and family health. This kind of certification requires passing an exam, 1,000 hours of teaching experience, plus direct experience caring for patients with the particular condition related to the specialization. For example, a nurse educator seeking certification in diabetes education might be a nurse at a hospital working with diabetic patients. The work may be a major or minor part of the nurse's regular work routine, or it may be volunteer work on the side.

EARNINGS

ACTUAL EARNINGS CAN VARY WIDELY, but the median annual salary for experienced nurse educators is about $85,000. Most salaries range between $75,000 and $95,000, depending on a variety of factors, such as location, years of experience in nursing and teaching, and any specializations within the field. Many in the academic field, start out as assistant professors. Their average salary is around $75,000, leaving plenty of room for growth.

It should be noted that like most teachers, nurse educators generally work only during the academic year. Summer teaching positions or any other summer jobs will be compensated separately on top of the base teacher's salary. Many nurse educators also earn extra income on the side by caring for patients.

Nurse educator jobs pay relatively well because of the advanced degree requirements. Like most occupations, the more education a nurse educator obtains, the greater the financial rewards. A master's degree garners a good salary, and a doctorate provides the opportunity for even more compensation.

Where a nurse educator is located affects earning potential. In many areas, nursing schools are offering more competitive salaries to attract qualified nurses into education. In other areas, caring for patients pays more than teaching. The type of institution is also a consideration. A for-profit school will pay more than a nonprofit. A nurse educator will earn more in a traditional environment than providing instruction online. The size of the institution, whether it is a hospital or a college, is a factor as well. Large institutions have the resources to pay more than smaller ones.

There are numerous ways to boost earnings in the nurse educator field. The first is to assume administrative or leadership responsibilities within the school. With the right training and experience, that could lead to a position as nurse education director or even dean. Those are high- level jobs with six figure salaries to match.

There are also specialized areas that pay more than general nursing education. Good paying jobs exist in the research field, for example. Nurse educators in research who have their work published in peer-reviewed journals are in a good position to command higher pay. Other possibilities for experienced nurse educators include working as an education consultant or serving as a spokesperson for public policy issues.

OPPORTUNITIES

THERE HAS NEVER BEEN A BETTER TIME to get started in a nurse educator career. Experts are projecting an almost 20 percent increase in the number of post-secondary nursing education jobs within the next decade. This is an extremely good job outlook compared to most other occupations.

The extreme demand is due primarily to a serious nursing shortage in the US. It is estimated that one million more nurses will be needed in just the next few years. According to the National League for Nursing (NLN), enrollment in nursing schools needs to increase by 30 percent in order to prepare that many nurses. The American Association of Colleges of Nursing (AACN) reports that 65,000 qualified applicants are turned away from nursing schools each year because there are not enough nurse educators to teach them!

Given the extreme shortage of nursing educators, it is an excellent time for current nurses to consider returning to school for an additional two or three years to prepare to transition into a teaching role. In fact, many government agencies, professional associations, and nonprofit organizations are actively campaigning to urge current nurses and even high school students to consider a career in nurse education. The shortage provides nurse educators excellent job prospects, a high level of job security, advancement opportunities, and the kind of flexibility clinical nurses do not typically have.

The growing demand in the nursing field is mostly being caused by the booming aging population. Older people generally need more healthcare services than those who are younger. The nursing population is also aging. Many job openings are being created by older nurses who are retiring. In the nurse education field specifically, an increase in the number of faculty retirements is expected to accelerate in the coming years leaving vacancies at most colleges and universities. This is good news for new nurse educators looking for their first teaching jobs.

While the biggest employer of nurse educators will continue to be educational institutions, there are other specialized areas that are growing fast. For example, pharmaceutical companies are starting to hire nurse educators. In this role, the nurse educator introduces and explains specific products or therapies within hospitals and physician networks. These companies have discovered that nurse educators have a much higher level of credibility than traditional drug reps and salespeople. They are able to quickly establish rapport and lay the groundwork for the kind of long lasting relationships that businesses need to thrive. They do not take the place of salespeople. They are teachers, providing instruction and fielding technical questions from the healthcare professionals who use the products.

GETTING STARTED

THE DEMAND FOR NURSE EDUCATORS is at an all-time high, so you may be surprised to find there is competition for the jobs you pursue. That is because, like in any other profession, employers are always searching for the best of the best candidates. Being qualified is just the prerequisite. Employers will look beyond your education and nursing experience for evidence of leadership qualities, respect in the field, and excellent teaching abilities. Make sure your résumé reflects these traits and that you share your philosophy of teaching during interviews.

Find ways to distinguish yourself before and during your job search. While still in school, seek out opportunities to become a teacher's assistant. It will provide valuable experience while providing you a platform to exhibit your talents. Look for other teaching experiences, such as mentoring or tutoring younger nursing students. Join the patient education team in a hospital or volunteer to instruct patients at a community clinic or nursing home. Become an adjunct or part-time clinical instructor in the area where you have the most expertise. There are often adjunct positions in areas that do not have many opportunities for teachers. The adjunct role is usually considered temporary, but it can lead to a full-time faculty position.

To increase your opportunities, throw a wider net. This is a flexible career with more possible work settings than you might imagine. Look for job titles and roles that call for your education and experience, but do not necessarily involve teaching nursing students directly. Examples include staff development officer, continuing education specialist, and public relations administrator.

Be sure to look beyond the hospital environment. A pharmaceutical company, a nonprofit health organization, or a research firm could employ you. In fact, jobs outside the healthcare field often offer better pay than hospitals. Also, look beyond your town. In some locations around the country, the need for nurse educators is not just great, it is urgent. Where that is the case, it means there are few candidates and therefore, less competition.

Networking is very important in the healthcare professions. In fact, it is how most nurse educators find jobs. Join professional nursing associations and attend their conferences. Attend career expos, join student groups in nursing school, and participate in work-study programs in as many hospitals as possible. In every situation that puts you in contact with potential colleagues and employers, go out of your way to network, make contacts, and stay in touch.

You can contact potential employers directly by calling the HR (human resources) departments in schools that have nurse training programs and hospitals. You can also search online. Nurse educator positions are posted on the general job sites, but there are also sites devoted to the healthcare field and nursing in particular. While you are online, check your professional associations. Most have job postings for members available on their sites.

Finally, consider earning a higher degree. The National League for Nursing has found that almost 70 percent of full-time nurse educators possess a master's degree while 25 percent hold a doctorate. Who do you think has a leg up on the competition for the best jobs? If you are not finding the job you want, it might be worth the investment to spend a little more time in school.

ASSOCIATIONS

■ **National Nursing Staff Development Organization**
www.nnsdo.org

■ **National League for Nursing**
www.nln.org

■ **American Association of Colleges of Nursing**
www.aacn.nche.edu

■ **Association for Nursing Professional Development**
http://www.anpd.org

PERIODICALS

■ **The Journal of Nursing Education**
www.healio.com/nursing/journals/jne

■ **Journal of Continuing Education in Nursing**
https://www.healio.com/nursing /journals/jcen

■ **Journal of Professional Nursing**
www.professionalnursing.org

WEBSITE

■ Health Occupations Students of America
http://www.hosa.org

www.ingramcontent.com/pod-product-compliance
Lightning Source LLC
Chambersburg PA
CBHW070522220526
45467CB00002B/799